# Tiny Miracle

## Everything You Need to Know About Caring for Your Premature Baby

**Ellen D. Brandon**

# Table of Contents

# INTRODUCTION

Mr. and Mrs. Smith were overjoyed when they found out they were expecting their first child. They had been together for many years and had always dreamed of starting a family. The pregnancy went smoothly, and Mrs. Smith was feeling great.

However, at 32 weeks, Mrs. Smith went into labor. The baby was born prematurely and weighed just 2 pounds. The doctors told Mr. and Mrs. Smith that the baby would need to stay in the NICU for several weeks.

Mr. and Mrs. Smith were devastated. They had never imagined that their child would be born so early. They were worried about the baby's health and were scared about what the future held.

The next few weeks were a blur for Mr. and Mrs. Smith. They spent every day at the hospital, holding their baby and praying for her health. The baby made slow progress, but she was eventually able to come home.

The first few months at home were challenging. The baby was small and fragile, and she needed a lot of care. Mr. and Mrs. Smith were exhausted, but they were determined to give their daughter the best possible care.

With time and love, the baby thrived. She grew bigger and stronger, and she started to develop her own personality. Mr. and Mrs. Smith were so happy to see their daughter healthy and happy.

The experience of having a premature baby was difficult, but it also brought Mr. and Mrs. Smith closer together. They learned that they could handle anything as long as they had each other. They are now the proud parents of a healthy and happy child, and they are grateful for every day they have with her.

Congratulations on the birth of your tiny miracle! Caring for a premature baby can be a daunting task, but with the right information and support, you can make it through this challenging time.

This book is designed to provide you with everything you need to know about caring for your premature baby. From the moment your baby is born, you will learn about the different stages of development and how to provide the best possible care. You will also learn about the different challenges that premature babies face and how to cope with them.

This book is not meant to replace the advice of your doctor or other healthcare professionals. However, it can provide you with a comprehensive overview of premature care and help you to feel more confident in your ability to care for your baby.

We hope that this book will be a valuable resource for you during this special time in your life.

# CHAPTER I

# What is a premature baby?

A baby who is born before 37 weeks of pregnancy is considered premature.The earlier a baby is born, the more likely they are to have health problems. Premature babies are often called preemies. Premature babies are often smaller and less developed than full-term babies, and they may have health problems. A baby's health is at greater risk the earlier it is born.

## Different Stages of Premature Development

**There are four main stages of premature development:**

**Late preterm**: Babies born between 34 and 36 weeks of pregnancy are considered late preterm. They are at a slightly higher risk of health problems than full-term babies, but most will go on to have healthy childhoods.

**Moderately preterm**: Babies born between 32 and 34 weeks of pregnancy are considered moderately preterm. They are at a higher risk of health problems than late preterm babies, but most will still have healthy childhoods.

**Very preterm**: Babies born before 32 weeks of pregnancy are considered very preterm. They are at the highest risk of health problems, including respiratory distress syndrome, brain hemorrhage, and necrotizing enterocolitis. Very preterm babies may need to stay in the neonatal intensive care unit (NICU) for several weeks or even months.

**Extremely preterm**: Babies born before 25 weeks of pregnancy are considered extremely preterm. They are the most vulnerable and have the highest risk of health problems. Extremely preterm babies often need to stay in the NICU for many months.

The development of premature babies can be delayed compared to full-term babies. For example, premature babies may reach developmental milestones, such as rolling over, sitting up, and walking, later than full-term babies. However, most premature babies will catch up to their peers by the time they reach school age.

# CHAPTER 2

# Causes of premature birth

There are some causes of premature birth

## 1. Infections

Infections are a leading cause of premature birth, accounting for an estimated 20-30% of all cases. Infections can occur in the mother's body, in the placenta, or in the amniotic fluid. They can be brought on by parasites, viruses, or bacteria.

**Types of infections that can cause premature birth**

- **Bacterial infections**

Bacterial infections are the most common type of infection that can cause premature birth. Some of the most common bacterial infections that can lead to preterm birth include:

* Group B Streptococcus (GBS)
* Streptococcus pyogenes (strep throat)

* Escherichia coli (E. coli)

* Listeria monocytogenes

* Neisseria gonorrhoeae (gonorrhea)

* Chlamydia trachomatis

- **Viral infections**

Viral infections are another common type of infection that can cause premature birth. Some of the most common viral infections that can lead to preterm birth include:

* Cytomegalovirus (CMV)

* Herpes simplex virus (HSV)

* Human papillomavirus (HPV)

* Rubella

* Zika virus

- **Parasitic infections**

Parasitic infections are less common than bacterial or viral infections, but they can also lead to premature birth. Some of the most common parasitic infections that can lead to preterm birth include:

* Toxoplasmosis

* Malaria

* Trichomoniasis

## How infections cause premature birth

Infections can cause premature birth in a number of ways. One way is by triggering an inflammatory response in the mother's body. This inflammatory response can lead to contractions of the uterus, which can eventually lead to preterm labor.

Infections can also damage the placenta, which is the organ that nourishes the baby during pregnancy. Damage to the placenta can reduce the amount of oxygen and nutrients that reach the baby, which can also lead to preterm labor.

Finally, infections can directly infect the baby, which can cause the baby to become sick and lead to preterm birth.

# How to prevent infections that cause premature birth

There are a number of things that pregnant women can do to help prevent infections that can cause premature birth. These include:

*** Getting regular prenatal care**
*** Getting vaccinated against common infections, such as GBS, HPV, and rubella**
*** Avoiding contact with sick people**
*** Practicing good hygiene, such as washing your hands frequently**

If you are pregnant and you think you may have an infection, it is important to see your doctor right away. Early treatment of infections can help to prevent preterm birth.

Overall, Infections are a leading cause of premature birth. There are a number of things that pregnant women can do to help prevent infections that can cause premature birth. If you are pregnant and you think you may have an infection, it is important to see your doctor right away. Early treatment of infections can help to prevent preterm birth.

# 2. Preeclampsia

Preeclampsia is a serious pregnancy complication that affects about 5-8% of pregnancies worldwide. It is characterized by high blood pressure, protein in the urine, and sometimes other symptoms such as headaches, vision problems, and swelling. Preeclampsia can cause serious health problems for both the mother and the baby, and it is one of the leading causes of preterm birth.

Preeclampsia is thought to be caused by a problem with the placenta, the organ that connects the mother to the baby and provides the baby with oxygen and nutrients. In preeclampsia, the placenta does not function properly and can damage the blood vessels in the mother's uterus. This can lead to high blood pressure, protein in the urine, and other symptoms.

Preeclampsia can occur at any time during pregnancy, but it is most common in the second half of pregnancy. It is also more common in first-time mothers, women who are pregnant with multiples, and women who have certain medical conditions such as diabetes or kidney disease.

Both the mother and the unborn child may face serious health issues as a result of preeclampsia. For the mother, preeclampsia can lead to seizures, stroke, and even death. For the baby, preeclampsia can cause preterm birth, low birth weight, and health problems such as brain hemorrhages and respiratory distress syndrome.

Preeclampsia cannot be cured, but it can be treated. Treatment for preeclampsia usually involves bed rest, medication to lower blood pressure, and delivery of the baby. If preeclampsia is mild, the baby may be able to stay in the womb until it is full-term. However, if preeclampsia is severe, the baby may need to be delivered early.

Premature birth is a major risk associated with preeclampsia. Premature babies are at risk for a number of health problems, including breathing problems, heart problems, brain problems, and eye problems. They may also have difficulty feeding and growing.

The best way to prevent preeclampsia is to get regular prenatal care. During prenatal care, your doctor will monitor your blood pressure and urine for signs of preeclampsia. If you are at risk for preeclampsia, your doctor may prescribe medication to help prevent it.

If you are diagnosed with preeclampsia, it is important to follow your doctor's instructions carefully. This may include taking medication, getting bed rest, and delivering the baby early. By following your doctor's instructions, you can help reduce the risk of complications for yourself and your baby.

**<u>Here are some additional information about preeclampsia:</u>**

* Preeclampsia is a serious condition, but it is usually treatable.
* The best way to prevent preeclampsia is to get regular prenatal care.
* If you are diagnosed with preeclampsia, it is important to follow your doctor's instructions carefully.
* With proper care, most women with preeclampsia and their babies go on to have healthy pregnancies and deliveries.

## 3. Placenta problems

An organ that grows inside the uterus during pregnancy is the placenta. It gets rid of waste and supplies the growing baby with oxygen and nutrients. Placental problems can affect the health of the baby and increase the risk of premature birth.

**There are many different types of placental problems, some of which can cause premature birth. These include:**

- **Placenta previa**: This is a condition where the placenta attaches low in the uterus, near or covering the cervix. Placenta previa can cause bleeding during pregnancy and can increase the risk of preterm birth.
- **Abruption of the placenta:** Before the baby is born, this is a condition in which the placenta separates from the uterine wall. Placental abruption can cause bleeding, and pain, and can be life-threatening for the mother and baby.
- **Placental insufficiency:** This is a condition where the placenta does not provide enough oxygen and nutrients to the baby. Placental insufficiency can cause the baby to grow slowly, and can increase the risk of preterm birth.
- **Placental infection**: This is an infection of the placenta. Placental infection can cause preterm birth, and can also increase the risk of health problems for the baby.

# 4. Multiple births

Multiple births are a major cause of premature birth. In fact, over 60% of twins and nearly all higher-order multiples are born before 37 weeks of gestation. The higher the number of fetuses in the pregnancy, the greater the risk for early birth.

There are a number of reasons why multiple births are more likely to result in premature birth. One reason is that the uterus can only stretch so much before it starts to put pressure on the cervix, which can lead to preterm labor. Additionally, multiple babies place a greater demand on the mother's body, which can lead to complications such as anemia, preeclampsia, and gestational diabetes. These complications can also increase the risk of preterm birth.

There are two main types of multiple births: identical twins and fraternal twins. Identical twins are formed when a single fertilized egg splits into two, while fraternal twins are formed when two separate eggs are fertilized by two separate sperm. Fraternal twins are less likely than identical twins to be born prematurely. This is because identical twins share the same placenta, which can lead to problems with blood flow and oxygen supply.

If a woman is carrying multiple babies and she experiences any signs of preterm labor, such as contractions, cramping, or vaginal bleeding, she should seek medical attention immediately. Early intervention can help to prevent premature birth and improve the chances of a healthy outcome for both mother and baby.

**Here are some additional information about multiple births and premature birth:**

* The rate of multiple births has been increasing in recent years, due in part to the use of fertility treatments such as in vitro fertilization (IVF).
* Premature birth is a serious condition that can lead to a number of health problems for babies, including low birth weight, respiratory problems, and developmental delays.
* There are a number of things that can be done to reduce the risk of premature birth in women who are carrying multiple babies, such as getting regular prenatal care and eating a healthy diet.
* If a woman is carrying multiple babies and she experiences any signs of preterm labor, such as contractions, cramping, or vaginal bleeding, she should seek medical attention immediately. Early intervention can help to prevent premature birth and improve the chances of a healthy outcome for both mother and baby.

# 5. Smoking

Smoking is one of the leading causes of premature birth. It is estimated that smoking increases the risk of preterm birth by 25-30%. Premature babies are at increased risk of health problems, such as low birth weight, respiratory problems, and developmental delays.

There are several ways that smoking can cause premature birth. Smoking can damage the placenta, which is the organ that provides oxygen and nutrients to the baby. Smoking can also increase the risk of preterm labor, which is the onset of contractions before 37 weeks of gestation.

If you are pregnant, it is important to quit smoking. There are many resources available to help you quit, such as your doctor, the American Lung Association, and the National Cancer Institute. The best thing you can do for your health and the health of your baby is to stop smoking.

**Here are some of the health risks associated with smoking during pregnancy:**

* Premature birth
* Low birth weight
* Stillbirth
* Sudden infant death syndrome (SIDS)
* Birth defects
* Respiratory problems
* Learning and behavioral problems

If you are pregnant and smoke, talk to your doctor about quitting. There are many resources available to help you quit, and quitting is the best thing you can do for your health and the health of your baby.

**Here are some tips for quitting smoking during pregnancy:**

* Let your doctor know that you need to stop.
* Set a quit date
* Tell your loved ones that you are stopping.
* Get rid of all cigarettes, cigars, and other tobacco products.
* Avoid situations where you are likely to smoke.

* Find healthy ways to cope with stress, such as exercise, relaxation techniques, or talking to a friend or therapist.
* Join a support group for people who are quitting smoking.

It's not easy to quit smoking, but it's worth it. If you are pregnant and smoke, quitting is the best thing you can do for your health and the health of your baby.

## 6. Drug use

Drug use during pregnancy can increase the risk of preterm birth. The following are some examples of drugs that can cause preterm birth:

* *Cocaine*: Cocaine can cause preterm labor, low birth weight, and birth defects.
* *Heroin*: Heroin can cause preterm labor, low birth weight, and birth defects.
* *Methamphetamine*: Methamphetamine can cause preterm labor, low birth weight, and birth defects.
* *Marijuana*: Marijuana can increase the risk of preterm labor and low birth weight.

* ***Alcohol***: Alcohol can cause fetal alcohol spectrum disorders (FASDs), which can include preterm birth, low birth weight, and birth defects.

* ***Tobacco***: Tobacco can cause preterm labor, low birth weight, and birth defects.

If you are pregnant and using drugs, it is important to get help. There are many resources available to help you get sober and stay sober during your pregnancy. Talk to your doctor about your drug use and they can help you find the resources you need.

**<u>Here are some of the ways that drug use can cause preterm birth</u>**:

- Drugs can damage the placenta, which is the organ that provides oxygen and nutrients to the fetus. This can lead to preterm labor and low birth weight.
- Drugs can increase the risk of infection, which can also lead to preterm labor.
- Drugs can cause the uterus to contract, which can lead to preterm labor.
- Drugs can affect the baby's development, which can lead to preterm birth.

If you are pregnant and using drugs, it is important to get help. There are many resources available to help you get sober and stay sober during your pregnancy. Talk to your doctor about your drug use and they can help you find the resources you need.

## 7. Alcohol use

Alcohol use during pregnancy is a leading cause of preterm birth.

There is no safe limit on how much alcohol a pregnant woman can consume. Even small amounts of alcohol can have a negative impact on the developing baby. Alcohol can enter the baby's bloodstream through the placenta. Numerous issues can result from this, including:

- Premature birth
- Low birth weight
- Birth defects
- Fetal alcohol spectrum disorders (FASDs)

FASDs are a gathering of conditions that can happen in children whose moms drank liquor during pregnancy.

FASDs can cause a wide range of physical and mental health problems, including:

* Growth and development delays

* Learning and behavioral problems

* Heart defects

* Vision and hearing problems

* Craniofacial abnormalities

If you are pregnant or planning to become pregnant, it is important to talk to your doctor about alcohol use. There is no need to completely stop drinking. Your doctor can help you develop a plan to safely stop drinking alcohol.

**Here are some examples of studies that have shown a link between alcohol use and preterm birth:**

- A study published in the journal "Alcoholism: Clinical and Experimental Research" in 2007 found that women who drank alcohol during pregnancy were more likely to deliver their babies preterm than women who did not drink alcohol.
- A study published in the journal "Pediatrics" in 2011 found that women who drank alcohol during pregnancy were more likely to

have babies with low birth weight than women who did not drink alcohol.

☐ A study published in the journal "Birth Defects Research Part A: Clinical and Molecular Teratology" in 2013 found that women who drank alcohol during pregnancy were more likely to have babies with birth defects than women who did not drink alcohol.

If you are pregnant or planning to become pregnant, Your doctor can help you develop a plan to safely stop drinking alcohol.

## 8. Chronic health conditions

Chronic health conditions can increase the risk of premature birth. Some of the most common chronic health conditions that can lead to premature birth include:

***Chronic high blood pressure***: High blood pressure can damage the placenta, which can lead to premature birth.

***Diabetes:*** Diabetes can cause the body to produce too much sugar, which can damage the placenta and increase the risk of premature birth.

**Chronic kidney disease**:. Chronic kidney disease can cause the body to retain fluid, which can put pressure on the uterus and increase the risk of premature birth.

**Anemia**:. A condition in which the body does not have enough healthy red blood cells is called Anemia. Red blood cells carry oxygen to the placenta, so anemia can reduce the amount of oxygen that reaches the baby, which can increase the risk of premature birth.

**Uterine fibroids**: Growths in the uterus that are not cancerous are known as uterine fibroids. Fibroids can sometimes put pressure on the cervix, which can increase the risk of premature birth.

**Infections:** Some infections, such as urinary tract infections and sexually transmitted infections, can increase the risk of premature birth.

**Pelvic inflammatory disease**: An infection that affects the female reproductive organs is called pelvic inflammatory disease. PID can damage the fallopian tubes and ovaries, which can increase the risk of premature birth.

**Placenta previa**: Placenta previa is a condition where the placenta covers part or the entirety of the cervix. Placenta previa can increase the risk of premature birth, as well as bleeding during pregnancy and childbirth.

**Placenta abruption**: A condition known as placenta abruption occurs when the placenta separates from the uterine wall before the baby is born. Placenta abruption can cause bleeding and can be life-threatening for both the mother and the baby.

If you have a chronic health condition, it is important to talk to your doctor about the risks of premature birth. Your doctor can help you manage your condition and take steps to reduce the risk of premature birth.

## 9. Age

Preterm birth is linked to maternal age. Women under the age of 20 and over the age of 40 are at an increased risk of delivering preterm. The risk of preterm birth increases with increasing maternal age and is highest for women over the age of 40.

There are a number of possible reasons why maternal age is a risk factor for preterm birth. One possibility is that older women are more likely to have health conditions that can lead to preterm birth, such as high blood pressure, diabetes, or obesity. Another possibility is that older women's bodies may not be able to support a pregnancy as well as younger women's bodies.

If you are concerned about your risk of preterm birth, talk to your doctor. There are a number of things that can be done to reduce your risk, and early diagnosis and treatment of preterm labor can help to improve the outcome for your baby.

Here are some additional information about the risk of preterm birth associated with maternal age:

- **Women under the age of 20:** Women under the age of 20 are at an increased risk of preterm birth for a number of reasons. One reason is that their bodies may not be fully developed, which can make it more difficult to carry a pregnancy to term. Another reason is that they may be more likely to have health conditions that can lead to preterm birth, such as anemia or low birth weight.
- **Women over the age of 40**: Women over the age of 40 are also at an increased risk of preterm birth. This is because their bodies may not be able to support a pregnancy as well as younger women's bodies. Additionally, older women are more likely to have health conditions that can lead to preterm birth, such as high blood pressure, diabetes, or obesity.

If you are a woman who is concerned about your risk of preterm birth, talk to your doctor. There are a number of things that you can do to reduce your risk, and early diagnosis and treatment of preterm labor can help to improve the outcome for your baby.

## 10.     Weight

**Underweight**: Women who are underweight before pregnancy are at an increased risk of preterm birth. This is because they may not have enough stored energy to support a healthy pregnancy.

**Overweight or obese**: Women who are overweight or obese are also at an increased risk of preterm birth. This is because they are more likely to have health conditions that can lead to preterm birth, such as gestational diabetes, high blood pressure, and preeclampsia.

**Rapid weight gain**: Women who gain too much weight during pregnancy are also at an increased risk of preterm birth. This is because rapid weight gain can put stress on the body and increase the risk of complications.

**Inadequate weight gain:** Women who do not gain enough weight during pregnancy are also at an increased risk of preterm birth. This is because the baby needs a certain amount of nutrients to grow and develop properly.

It is important to note that weight is just one factor that can contribute to preterm birth. Other factors, such as genetics, age, and health conditions, can also play a role. However, by maintaining a healthy weight before and during pregnancy, women can help reduce their risk of preterm birth.

If you are concerned about your weight or your risk of preterm birth, talk to your doctor. They can help you develop a plan to reduce your risk and have a healthy pregnancy.

## 11.     Race or ethnicity

Race and ethnicity are known to be risk factors for preterm birth. In the United States, black women are 2.5 times more likely to have a preterm birth than white women. American Indians/Alaska Natives and Hispanics are also at an increased risk of preterm birth.

**There are a number of factors that may contribute to the racial and ethnic disparities in preterm birth. These factors include:**

- *Socioeconomic factors*:  Black and Hispanic women are more likely to live in poverty and have less access to healthcare. These factors can contribute to preterm birth by increasing the risk of chronic health conditions, such as obesity and diabetes, which are also risk factors for preterm birth.

- *Healthcare access*: Black and Hispanic women are less likely to have access to prenatal care, which can help to identify and manage risk factors for preterm birth.
- *Social determinants of health*: . Black and Hispanic women are more likely to experience stress and trauma, which can increase the risk of preterm birth.
- *Genetic factors*: There may be genetic factors that contribute to the racial and ethnic disparities in preterm birth. However, more studies are to be carried out in this area.

It is important to note that these are just some of the factors that may contribute to the racial and ethnic disparities in preterm birth. There is no single cause of preterm birth, and it is likely that a combination of factors plays a role.

*There are a number of things that can be done to reduce the risk of preterm birth for all women, regardless of race or ethnicity. These include:*

a. ***Access to quality prenatal care***: . All women should have access to quality prenatal care, which can help to identify and manage risk factors for preterm birth.

b. ***Healthy lifestyle choices:*** Women can reduce their risk of preterm birth by making healthy lifestyle choices, such as eating a healthy diet, exercising regularly, and not smoking or drinking alcohol during pregnancy.

c. ***Support***: Women who are at risk of preterm birth may benefit from support from friends, family, and healthcare providers. This support can help them to cope with stress and make healthy lifestyle choices.

By addressing the factors that contribute to preterm birth, we can help to reduce the racial and ethnic disparities in this serious condition.

## 12. Medical history

Women with a history of premature birth are at an increased risk of having another premature birth. This is because the body may be more likely to go into labor early due to changes in the cervix or uterus.

## ✓ Uterine problems

Uterine problems can be a cause of premature birth. Some of the most common uterine problems that can lead to preterm birth include:

* Uterine fibroids:  Fibroids are non-cancerous growths that can develop in the uterus. They are very common, affecting up to 80% of women by the time they reach menopause. Fibroids can cause the uterus to become enlarged and misshapen, which can put pressure on the cervix and make it more likely to dilate prematurely.

* Cervical insufficiency:  Cervical insufficiency is a condition in which the cervix (the neck of the uterus) is weak or unable to support the weight of the growing baby. This can lead to the cervix dilating and opening prematurely, which can cause preterm birth.

* Uterine malformations: Uterine malformations are birth defects that can affect the shape or size of the uterus. Some types of uterine malformations can make it more difficult for the baby to grow and develop in the uterus, which can increase the risk of preterm birth.

* Uterine infection: An infection of the uterus can cause inflammation and irritation, which can lead to preterm birth. Some of the most common types of uterine infections that can lead to preterm birth include:

*Bacterial vaginosis*

*Trichomoniasis*

*Chlamydia*

*Gonorrhea*

*Human papillomavirus (HPV)*

If you have any of the risk factors for preterm birth, it is important to talk to your doctor.

If you experience any symptoms of preterm labor, such as contractions, cramping, or vaginal bleeding, it is important to seek medical attention right away. Early treatment can help to prevent preterm birth and improve the chances of a healthy baby.

## 13. Trauma

Trauma can be a cause of premature birth. It can be physical trauma, such as a car accident or a fall, or it can be emotional trauma, such as the death of a loved one or a natural disaster. Trauma can cause the body to release stress hormones, which can lead to preterm labor.

**Here are some examples of how trauma can lead to premature birth:**

A woman who is in a car accident and experiences physical trauma may go into preterm labor.

A woman who is the victim of domestic violence may go into preterm labor due to the emotional trauma she experiences.

A woman who has experienced a miscarriage or stillbirth in the past may be more likely to go into preterm labor due to the emotional trauma of those experiences.

A woman who is living in a war zone or other dangerous environment may be more likely to go into preterm labor due to the stress of living in a dangerous place.

If you have experienced trauma, it is important to talk to your doctor about the risks of preterm birth. There are things you can do to reduce your risk, such as getting regular prenatal care and taking care of your mental health.

**Signs and symptoms of premature labor**

When labor starts before 37 weeks of pregnancy, it is called preterm labor. It is a serious condition that can lead to health problems for the baby and mother.

There are many signs and symptoms of preterm labor. Some of the most common include:

✓ **Contractions:** The contraction of the uterine muscles is known as a contracture. They can be felt as a tightening or hardening of the belly. Contractions may be regular or irregular, and they may be painful or painless.

✓ **Pelvic pressure**. Some women may feel pressure in their pelvis or lower abdomen as if the baby is pushing down.

✓ Diarrhea. Some women may experience diarrhea before preterm labor.

✓ **Vaginal discharge**. The vaginal discharge of some women might change. it may be watery, bloody, or mucus-like.

✓ **Rupture of membranes**. The rupture of membranes is when the amniotic sac breaks. This can cause a woman to leak fluid from her vagina.

If you experience any of these signs or symptoms, it is important to call your doctor right away. Preterm labor can be stopped with treatment, but it is important to get treatment as soon as possible.

**Here are some examples of preterm labor:**

* A woman who is 34 weeks pregnant starts to have regular contractions every 5 minutes.
* A woman who is 36 weeks pregnant starts to leak fluid from her vagina.
* A woman who is 35 weeks pregnant has a sudden onset of diarrhea and pelvic pressure.

If you experience any of these signs or symptoms, it is important to call your doctor right away. Preterm labor can be stopped with treatment, but it is important to get treatment as soon as possible.

# CHAPTER 3

# Complications of premature birth

Premature birth is the birth of a baby before 37 weeks of pregnancy. Premature babies are at risk for a number of complications, including:

1. **Respiratory distress syndrome (RDS)**: RDS is a lung condition that occurs when the lungs are not fully developed. It is the most common complication of premature birth, affecting about 60% of babies born before 32 weeks of pregnancy. RDS is caused by a lack of surfactant, a substance that helps keep the lungs inflated. Symptoms of RDS include rapid breathing, grunting, and cyanosis (a bluish tint to the skin). Treatment for RDS includes giving the baby oxygen and surfactant medication.

2. **Bronchopulmonary dysplasia (BPD)**. BPD is a chronic lung disease that can occur in premature babies who have had RDS. BPD is caused by damage to the lungs that occurs during RDS. Symptoms of BPD include persistent coughing, wheezing, and shortness of breath. Treatment for BPD may include oxygen therapy, medications, and respiratory support.

3. **Intraventricular hemorrhage (IVH)**. Bleeding in the brain that can occur in premature babies is called IVH. IVH is more common in babies born before 32 weeks of pregnancy. Symptoms of IVH may include seizures, vomiting, and poor feeding. Treatment for IVH may include medication, surgery, and supportive care.

4. **Necrotizing enterocolitis (NEC).** NEC is a serious inflammation of the intestines that can occur in premature babies. NEC is more common in babies born before 32 weeks of pregnancy. Symptoms of NEC may include abdominal distension, vomiting, and bloody stools. Treatment for NEC may include surgery, antibiotics, and supportive care.

5. **Neonatal sepsis**. Sepsis is a blood infection that can occur in premature babies. Sepsis is more common in babies born before 32 weeks of pregnancy. Symptoms of sepsis may include fever, chills, and poor feeding. Treatment for sepsis includes antibiotics and supportive care.

6. **Patent ductus arteriosus (PDA).** PDA is a heart defect that can occur in premature babies. PDA is caused by a hole in the wall between two of the heart's main arteries. Symptoms of PDA may include rapid breathing, poor feeding, and sweating. Treatment for PDA may include surgery or medication.

7. **Retinopathy of prematurity (ROP).** ROP is a condition that can affect the eyes of premature babies. ROP is brought about by unusual vein development in the retina, the light-delicate tissue at the rear of the eye. Symptoms of ROP may include poor vision and eye problems. Treatment for ROP may include laser surgery or cryotherapy.

**Premature babies are also at risk for long-term health problems, such as:**

*Cerebral palsy*: Cerebral palsy is a group of disorders that can cause problems with movement, muscle tone, and posture. Cerebral palsy can occur in babies born preterm or at full term.

* **Breathing problems**: Premature babies' lungs are not fully developed, so they may have difficulty breathing. They may need to be put on a ventilator to help them breathe.

* **Infections**: Because their immune systems are not fully developed, premature infants are more susceptible to infections. They may need to be given antibiotics to prevent or treat infections.

* **Brain problems:** Premature babies are at risk of brain injuries from a lack of oxygen or bleeding in the brain. These injuries can lead to cerebral palsy, learning disabilities, and other problems.

* **Eye problems**: Premature babies' eyes are not fully developed, so they may be more likely to develop eye problems such as retinopathy of prematurity. This condition can lead to blindness.

Growth problems: Premature babies may not grow as quickly as full-term babies. They may also be more likely to have low birth weight and be underweight for their age.

* **Learning disabilities** Premature babies are at increased risk for learning disabilities, such as dyslexia and attention deficit hyperactivity disorder (ADHD). Learning disabilities can occur due to damage to the brain or the nervous system.

The severity of the complications of premature birth can vary depending on the gestational age of the baby and the severity of the prematurity. With advances in medical care, many premature babies are able to survive and thrive. However, premature babies are still at risk for a number of health problems, both short-term and long-term.

# CHAPTER 4

# Preventing Premature Birth

If you are pregnant and you are concerned about your risk of premature birth, talk to your doctor. There are treatments that can help reduce your risk and help your baby stay healthy.

**Here are some examples of how you can reduce your risk of premature birth:**

✓ ***Reach a healthy weight prior to becoming pregnant and maintain that weight throughout the process***. Being overweight or obese increases your risk of premature birth. Aim to gain a healthy amount of weight during pregnancy, which is about 25 to 35 pounds for women who start out at a healthy weight.

✓ _**Try not to smoke, drink liquor, use road medications, or misuse**_

_**physician recommended drugs.**_ Smoking, drinking alcohol, and using drugs can all increase your risk of premature birth. Stopping smoking and keeping away from liquor and medications are everything things you can manage to safeguard your child's wellbeing.

As soon as you think you might be pregnant, go to your first prenatal care appointment. Prenatal care can help identify and treat any health problems that could increase your risk of premature birth. It's also a good time to talk to your doctor about ways to reduce your risk of premature birth.

✓ _**Get treated for chronic health conditions, like high blood pressure,**_

_**diabetes, depression, and thyroid problems**_. Chronic health conditions can increase your risk of premature birth. Getting these conditions treated can help reduce your risk.

✓ _**Eating a healthy diet**_

Eating a healthy diet is important for everyone, but it is especially important for pregnant women. A healthy diet can help to prevent a variety of pregnancy complications, including premature birth.

A premature birth is one that takes place prior to 37 weeks of pregnancy. It is a leading cause of death and disability in newborns. There are many factors that can contribute to premature birth, including infection, chronic health conditions, and poor nutrition.

A healthy diet during pregnancy can help to reduce the risk of premature birth by providing the baby with the nutrients it needs to grow and develop properly. A healthy diet also helps to maintain the mother's health and prevent complications such as anemia, gestational diabetes, and preeclampsia.

**The following are some important nutrients for pregnant women:**

* *Folic acid*:  Folic acid is fundamental for forestalling brain tube absconds, for example, spina bifida. Pregnant women should get 400 micrograms of folic acid daily.
* *Iron*: Iron is needed to make red blood cells, which carry oxygen to the baby. Pregnant women should get 27 milligrams of iron daily.
* *Calcium*: Calcium is needed for building strong bones and teeth in the baby. Pregnant women should get 1000 milligrams of calcium daily.
* *Vitamin D:* Vitamin D helps the body absorb calcium. Pregnant women should get 10 micrograms of vitamin D daily.

In addition to getting enough of these nutrients, pregnant women should also avoid certain foods and drinks that can increase the risk of premature birth. These include:

* *Unpasteurized milk and cheese*
* *Raw fish*
* *Alcohol*
* *Caffeine*
* *Tobacco*

By eating a healthy diet and avoiding harmful substances, pregnant women can help to reduce the risk of premature birth and give their babies the best possible start in life.

**Here are some additional tips for eating a healthy diet during pregnancy:**

* Eat plenty of fruits and vegetables. Fruits and vegetables are packed with vitamins, minerals, and fiber, which are all important for a healthy pregnancy.

* Choose whole grains over refined grains. Entire grains give more fiber and supplements than refined grains.

* Eat lean protein sources. Lean protein sources include fish, chicken, beans, and tofu.

* Limit unhealthy fats. Unhealthy fats, such as saturated and trans fats, can increase the risk of preterm birth.

* Drink plenty of water. Water is essential for staying hydrated and preventing constipation.

If you have any questions about what to eat during pregnancy, talk to your doctor or a registered dietitian. They can help you create a healthy eating plan that is right for you and your baby.

## ✓ Getting enough exercise

Getting enough exercise during pregnancy can help to prevent premature birth. Exercise helps to strengthen the muscles and bones, improve circulation, and reduce stress. It can also help to control weight gain, which is a risk factor for preterm birth.

The Centers for Disease Control and Prevention (CDC) recommends that pregnant women get at least 30 minutes of moderate-intensity aerobic activity most days of the week. Moderate-intensity aerobic activity includes activities such as brisk walking, swimming, and biking.

When you're pregnant, it's important to talk to your doctor before starting any new exercise program..Your doctor can help you to create a safe and effective exercise plan that is right for you.

**Here are a few methods for practicing securely during pregnancy**:

* Begin slowly and gradually increase your workout intensity and duration.
* Pay attention to your body and stop when you're in pain.
* Get plenty of fluids to stay hydrated.
* Try not to practice in blistering climate or then again assuming you have any wellbeing concerns.

Exercise is a great way to stay healthy during pregnancy and can help to prevent premature birth. If you have any questions about exercising during pregnancy, talk to your doctor.

**Here are some of the benefits of exercise during pregnancy**:

* *Helps to control weight gain*

* *Reduces the risk of gestational diabetes*

* *Improves mood and sleep*

* *Strengthens the muscles and bones*

* *Improves circulation*

* *Reduces stress*

* *Helps the body to recover after childbirth*

If you are pregnant and are not used to exercising, start slowly and gradually increase the intensity and duration of your workouts. It is important to listen to your body and stop if you feel pain. Stay hydrated by drinking plenty of fluids. Avoid exercising in hot weather or if you have any health concerns.

Exercise is a great way to stay healthy during pregnancy and can help to prevent premature birth. If you have any questions about exercising during pregnancy, talk to your doctor.

## ✓ *Getting enough sleep*

Sleep deprivation is another factor that has been linked to an increased risk of preterm birth. Studies have shown that women who get less than

7 hours of sleep per night are more likely to deliver their babies prematurely than women who get 7 or more hours of sleep per night.

The exact mechanism by which sleep deprivation increases the risk of preterm birth is not fully understood. However, it is thought that sleep deprivation may lead to changes in hormone levels and inflammation, which can both contribute to preterm labor.

**There are a number of things that pregnant women can do to improve their sleep quality and reduce their risk of preterm birth. These include:**

* Going to bed and waking up at the same time each day, even on weekends
* Creating a relaxing bedtime routine
* Avoiding caffeine and alcohol before bed
* Making sure the bedroom is dark, quiet, and cool
* Exercising regularly, but not too close to bedtime
* Seeing a doctor if you are having trouble sleeping

Getting enough sleep is an important part of a healthy pregnancy. By following the tips above, you can improve your sleep quality and reduce your risk of preterm birth.

*Here are some additional tips for getting a good night's sleep during pregnancy:*

* Avoid napping during the day. This can make it harder to fall asleep at night.
* Make sure your bedroom is dark, quiet, and cool.
* Use a comfortable mattress and pillows.
* Avoid watching TV or using electronic devices in bed. The blue light emitted from these devices can interfere with sleep.
* If you can't fall asleep after 20 minutes, get out of bed and do something relaxing until you feel tired.
* Talk to your doctor if you have trouble sleeping. There may be an underlying medical condition that is affecting your sleep.

✓ ___Managing stress___

There are a number of factors that can increase the risk of premature birth, including stress.

Studies have shown that stress can increase the risk of premature birth in a number of ways. Stress can cause changes in the body that can make it more likely for the baby to be born early. For example, stress can increase the production of hormones that can cause the uterus to contract. Stress can also weaken the cervix, which is the opening to the uterus. A weak cervix can make it more likely for the cervix to open early, which can lead to premature birth.

If you are pregnant and are feeling stressed, it is important to talk to your doctor. They can help you develop a plan to manage your stress and reduce the risk of premature birth.

**Here are some additional tips for managing stress during pregnancy:**

- Identify your stressors. The first step to managing stress is to identify what is causing it. Once you know what your stressors are, you can start to develop strategies for dealing with them.

- Take breaks. When you're feeling stressed, it's important to take breaks throughout the day. Get up and move around, or do something relaxing like reading or listening to music.

- Talk to someone. If you're struggling to cope with stress, talk to someone you trust. This could be a friend, family member, therapist, or other healthcare provider. Talking about your feelings can help you feel better and develop coping mechanisms.

- Protect yourself from infections. Infections, such as urinary tract infections or sexually transmitted infections, can increase your risk of premature birth. Practice good hygiene and get regular checkups to help prevent infections.

- Reduce your stress. Stress can increase your risk of premature birth. Find healthy ways to manage stress, such as yoga, meditation, or spending time with loved ones.

Stand by something like year and a half between conceiving an offspring and getting pregnant once more.

Having a baby too soon after a previous premature birth increases your risk of having another premature birth. Wait at least 18 months between pregnancies to give your body time to heal.

By following these tips, you can help reduce your risk of premature birth and give your baby the best possible start in life.

# CHAPTER 5

## Premature Babies and Autism

## What is Autism?

Autism Spectrum Disorder (ASD) is a formative incapacity that can cause critical social, correspondence, and conduct difficulties. People with ASD may communicate, interact, behave, and learn in ways that are distinct from the majority of other people, but there is typically nothing about their appearance that distinguishes them from other people.

People with ASD can be gifted or severely challenged in their learning, thinking, and problem-solving abilities. Certain individuals with ASD need a ton of help in their day to day routines; Others require less While some people with ASD can live independently, others require ongoing assistance.

Autism is not caused by anything that a parent does or does not do during pregnancy or after the child is born. Although the precise cause of ASD is unknown, it is likely brought on by a combination of environmental and genetic factors.

There is no one-size-fits-all treatment for ASD. The best approach for each person will vary depending on their individual needs and abilities. Some common treatments for ASD include:

* **Applied behavior analysis (ABA)**: ABA is a type of therapy that helps people with ASD learn new skills and behaviors.

***Language training**: Language instruction can assist individuals with ASD further develop their relational abilities.

* **Occupational therapy**: Occupational therapy can help people with ASD learn how to do activities of daily living, such as dressing, eating, and using the bathroom.

* **Social skills training**: Social skills training can help people with ASD learn how to interact with others in a more appropriate way.

Early intervention is important for people with ASD. Early intervention can help people with ASD learn new skills and behaviors, and it can also help them reach their full potential.

**Here are some examples of people with autism:**

1. Temple **Grandin** is a world-renowned autism advocate and animal behaviorist. She is the writer of a few books, including "The Autistic Brain" and "Thinking in Pictures."
2. **Dan Aykroyd** is an entertainer, jokester, and author. He is best known for his roles in Ghostbusters and "Saturday Night Live"
3. **Greta Thunberg** is a Swedish environmental activist. She is known for her work to raise awareness about climate change.

These are just a few examples of the many people with autism who have made significant contributions to society. Autism is a spectrum, and each person with autism is unique. With early intervention and support, people with autism can live full and productive lives.

## Premature Babies and Autism

There is a link between premature birth and autism spectrum disorder (ASD). The earlier a baby is born, the higher the risk of developing

ASD. For example, a study published in the journal Pediatrics found that children born at 22 to 27 weeks of gestation had nearly four times the risk of developing ASD than full-term infants born between 39 and 41 weeks.

The exact cause of the link between premature birth and ASD is not fully understood, but it is thought to be due to a combination of genetic and environmental factors. Premature babies are more likely to experience brain injuries and other complications that can increase the risk of ASD.

Additionally, premature babies may be exposed to more environmental toxins and pollutants that can also increase the risk of ASD.

There is no cure for ASD, but early intervention can help improve the outcomes for children with the disorder. Early intervention programs can help children learn communication, social skills, and other skills that can help them succeed in school and in life.

**Here are some examples of how premature birth can increase the risk of autism:**

* Babies born before 32 weeks of gestation are more likely to have brain injuries that can lead to autism.

* Premature babies are more likely to be exposed to infections that can increase the risk of autism.

* Premature babies are more likely to be exposed to environmental toxins that can increase the risk of autism.

If you have a premature baby, it is important to talk to your doctor about the risk of autism. Early intervention can help improve the outcomes for children with autism.

# CHAPTER 6

# Premature babies vs full-term babies

Premature babies are born before 37 weeks of pregnancy, while full-term babies are born after 37 weeks. Premature babies are at higher risk for health problems than full-term babies, including respiratory problems, feeding problems, and developmental delays.

*Here are some of the key differences between premature and full-term babies:*

i. <u>Gestational age</u>: Premature babies are born before 37 weeks of pregnancy, while full-term babies are born after 37 weeks.

ii. <u>Weight:</u> Premature babies are typically much smaller than full-term babies. The average weight of a full-term baby is 7 pounds, while the average weight of a premature baby is 5 pounds or less.

iii. <u>Body fat:</u> Premature babies have less body fat than full-term babies. This can make them more susceptible to hypothermia (low body temperature).

iv. <u>Organ development</u>: Premature babies' organs are not fully developed. This can lead to health problems, such as respiratory problems, feeding problems, and developmental delays.

v. <u>NICU care:</u> Premature babies often need to stay in the neonatal intensive care unit (NICU) for care. The NICU is a special unit in the hospital that provides care for premature and sick babies.

The health of premature babies can vary depending on their gestational age and birth weight. Babies born at 34 weeks of pregnancy are at lower risk for health problems than babies born at 28 weeks of pregnancy. Babies born at 28 weeks of pregnancy are considered to be extremely premature and are at the highest risk for health problems.

With the help of modern medicine, many premature babies go on to live healthy lives. However, it is important to be aware of the risks associated with premature birth so that you can get the best possible care for your baby.

# CHAPTER 7

# How to take care of your premature child in the NICU

The NICU is a special unit in the hospital where premature babies can receive the care they need. If your baby is born premature, they will be taken to the neonatal intensive care unit (NICU). The NICU staff is highly trained and experienced in caring for premature babies.

Parents of premature babies often feel scared and overwhelmed. They may worry about their baby's health and whether they will be able to go home. The NICU staff can provide support and education to help parents cope with this difficult time.

Caring for a premature baby in the NICU can be a challenging and emotional experience for parents. However, there are many things you can do to help your baby during this time.

**Here are some tips for caring for your premature baby in the NICU:**

1. **Get to know the NICU staff.** The NICU staff are experts in caring for premature babies. They will be able to answer your questions and provide you with support.
2. **Learn about your baby's condition.** The more you know about your baby's condition, the better equipped you will be to care for them. The NICU staff can provide you with information about your baby's medical needs.
3. **Be involved in your baby's care.** The NICU staff will encourage you to be involved in your baby's care as much as possible. This

will help you bond with your baby and make the NICU experience less stressful.

4. **Hold your baby as much as possible**. Skin-to-skin contact is beneficial for premature babies. It helps keep their breathing, temperature, and heart rate in check. It additionally assists with lessening pressure and advance holding.

5. **Breastfeed your baby if possible**. Bosom milk is the best sustenance for untimely infants. It provides them with antibodies and other nutrients that help them fight infection and develop properly.

6. **Be patient.** Caring for a premature baby can be a long and challenging process. Being patient and taking things one day at a time are essential.

With the help of the NICU staff and your own support network, you can provide your premature baby with the care they need to thrive.

# CHAPTER 8

# Taking your premature baby home

The day my baby was born, I was so excited to finally meet him. But my excitement quickly turned to worry when the doctors told me he was premature. He was only 36 weeks old, and he weighed just 4 pounds.

The doctors said that he would need to stay in the neonatal intensive care unit (NICU) for a few weeks. I was heartbroken, but I knew that he was in the best place pThey took such great consideration of my child. They were always there to answer my questions and to offer support.

After a few weeks, my baby was finally strong enough to come home. I was so happy to finally have him home with me. However, I also felt a little bit of fear. I had no idea what to anticipate.

The doctors gave me a lot of information about how to care for my premature baby. They told me to keep him warm, to feed him every 3 hours, and to watch for any signs of infection.

I took care of my baby around the clock. I fed him, I changed his diapers, and I held him close. I was so grateful to have him home with me.

My baby is now 6 months old, and he is doing great. He is healthy and happy. I am so proud of him.

Taking a premature baby home can be a daunting task, but it is also an amazing experience. It is a time to bond with your child and to celebrate their arrival. With the help of doctors and nurses, you will be able to provide your baby with the care they need to thrive.

Taking your premature baby home can be a daunting task, but it is also an exciting time. After spending weeks or even months in the neonatal intensive care unit (NICU), you are finally able to bring your little one home.

There are a few things you need to do to prepare for your baby's homecoming. First, make sure you have a safe and comfortable place for your baby to sleep. A bassinet or crib in your bedroom is ideal, as this will allow you to keep a close eye on your baby.

You will also need to make sure your home is safe for a premature baby. This means removing any potential hazards, such as sharp objects, cords, and chemicals. You should also avoid smoking in your home, as this can be harmful to your baby's health.

Once your home is safe, you can start thinking about feeding your baby. If your baby is able to breastfeed, this is the best option. However, if your baby is not able to breastfeed or if you choose not to breastfeed, you will need to formula feed.

Your baby's doctor will be able to give you more specific instructions on how to feed your baby. In general, premature babies need to be fed more often than full-term babies. They may also need to be fed with a special type of formula.

In addition to feeding, you will also need to keep your baby warm. Premature babies are not able to regulate their body temperature as well as full-term babies. This means you will need to dress your baby warmly and keep the room temperature at a comfortable level.

Finally, you will need to be prepared for any medical problems that your baby may experience. Premature babies are at risk for a number of health problems, including respiratory problems, jaundice, and infections. It is important to be aware of these risks and to seek medical attention if your baby experiences any problems.

Taking your premature baby home can be a challenge, but it is also a rewarding experience. With proper care and support, your baby will thrive and grow into a healthy and happy child.

**Here are some additional tips for taking your premature baby home:**

* Get plenty of rest. You will need your energy to care for your baby.
* Ask for help from family and friends. Don't be afraid to ask for help with things like cooking, cleaning, and childcare.

* Join a group that helps parents of premature children. This can be an extraordinary method for interfacing with different guardians who comprehend what you are going through.

* Take care of yourself. Make sure to eat healthy, get enough exercise, and take some time for yourself each day.

# CHAPTER 9

# Bonding with Your Premature Baby

Bonding with your premature baby is important for both you and your child. It helps to create a close relationship and can have a positive impact on your baby's development.

**There are many ways to bond with your premature baby, even if they are in the NICU. Here are a few ideas:**

**Holding and touching your baby.** This is one of the most important things you can do to bond with your baby. Even if they are small and fragile, they can feel your touch and it will help them to feel safe and secure.

**Talking to your baby.** Talk to your baby about your day, what you are doing, and how much you love them. Even if they can't understand your words, they can hear your voice and it will help them to feel connected to you.

**Singing to your baby**. The sound of your voice is soothing and calming for your baby. Sing to them their favorite songs or make up your own melodies.

**Reading to your baby**. Reading to your baby is a great way to bond and expose them to language. Choose books that are bright and colorful and that have simple stories.

**Massaging your baby**. Gentle massage can help to relax your baby and promote their development. Use a light touch and focus on their back, arms, and legs.

**Spending time with your baby**. Even if you can't hold your baby, you can still bond with them by spending time in their room. Talk to them, sing to them, and read to them. Just being close to them will help to create a strong bond.

Bonding with your premature baby may take some time and effort, but it is worth it. The benefits of bonding are long-lasting and can help your baby to thrive.

Here are some additional tips for bonding with your premature baby and supporting your baby's development

* Be patient. It may take some time for your baby to adjust to being outside the womb. Be patient and understanding, and don't be afraid to ask for help from the NICU staff.
*Get down on the floor and play with your baby. They will learn how to interact with the world around them thanks to this.
*Talk about what you're doing as you're doing it. Your baby will learn more about the world around them.
*Sing songs and makeup rhymes. Your baby's language development will be aided by this.

*Read books and magazines. Your baby will learn more about the world around them thanks to this.

*Take your baby for walks and outings. This will help them experience new things and learn about their surroundings.

*Expose your baby to different cultures and languages. This will help them develop a global perspective.

*Encourage your baby to explore and experiment. This will help them learn and grow.

*Be patient and loving. Every day, your baby grows and learns new things. Show them how much you care by being patient with them.

* Trust your instincts. You know your baby best. If you think something is wrong, don't be afraid to speak up.

* Deal with yourself. During this time, it's important to take care of yourself physically and emotionally. Make sure you get enough sleep, eat healthy, and give yourself time to relax.

Bonding with your premature baby can be a challenging but rewarding experience. By following these tips, you can help to create a strong and lasting bond with your child.

# CHAPTER 10

## Common challenges of caring for a premature baby

Before 37 weeks of pregnancy, a baby is delivered prematurely. They are often smaller and less developed than full-term babies, and they may have health challenges that require special care.

**Some of the common challenges of caring for a premature baby include:**

- **Breathing problems:** Premature babies' lungs may not be fully developed, which can lead to breathing problems such as respiratory distress syndrome (RDS). RDS is a condition that causes the lungs to become inflamed and stiff, making it difficult for the baby to breathe.

- **Feeding problems**: Premature babies' digestive systems may not be fully developed, which can make it difficult for them to eat and digest food. They may also have trouble sucking and swallowing, which can lead to weight loss and other health problems.

- **Temperature regulation:** Premature babies' bodies are not yet able to regulate their temperature as well as full-term babies. This can lead to hypothermia (low body temperature) or hyperthermia (high body temperature).

- **Infection**. Premature babies are more susceptible to infection than full-term babies. This is because they do not yet have fully developed immune systems.

- **NICU stay**: Premature babies often need to stay in the neonatal intensive care unit (NICU) for several weeks or even months. This can be a difficult time for parents, who may not be able to hold or touch their baby as much as they would like.

Despite the challenges, most premature babies go on to live healthy lives. With the right care and support, they can reach their full potential.

***Instances of how these challenges can impact a premature baby and their family:***

* A baby with RDS may need to be placed on a ventilator, which helps them breathe. This can be a frightening experience for parents, who may feel helpless as their baby struggles to breathe.
* A baby with feeding problems may need to be fed through a tube. This can be difficult for parents, who may feel like they are not able to provide for their baby's basic needs.
* A baby with temperature regulation problems may need to be kept in a special incubator. This can make it difficult for parents to hold and cuddle their baby.
* A baby with an infection may need to be treated with antibiotics. This can be a long and difficult process, and it can be scary for parents to see their baby so sick.

* A baby who needs to stay in the NICU for a long time may miss out on important bonding time with their parents. This can be a difficult experience for both the baby and the parents.

Despite the challenges, most premature babies go on to live healthy lives. With the right care and support, they can reach their full potential.

# CHAPTER 11

# Caring for Yourself As You Care For Your Premature Baby

Caring for a premature baby can be a very challenging experience. It is essential to keep in mind that you are not alone and that numerous resources are available to assist you. Here are some tips for caring for yourself as you care for your premature baby:

**<u>Get enough rest</u>.** This is especially important if you are also a new parent. Try to get as much sleep as possible, even if it means napping during the day.

**<u>Eat a healthy diet</u>.** Eating nutritious foods will help you stay strong and healthy so that you can care for your baby.

**<u>Stay hydrated</u>.**It is important to drink plenty of fluids, especially water.

**<u>Take breaks</u>.** It is important to take breaks from caring for your baby, even if it is just for a few minutes. Take a bath, read a book, or go for a walk.

**Talk to someone**. Talking to someone about how you are feeling can help you cope with the stress of caring for a premature baby. This could be a companion, relative, specialist, or care group.

**Ask for help**. Do not be afraid to ask for help from your partner, family, friends, or healthcare providers. They can help you with tasks such as cooking, cleaning, and taking care of your other children.

It is also important to remember to take care of your emotional well-being. It is normal to feel a range of emotions after the birth of a premature baby, such as sadness, anxiety, anger, and guilt. If you are struggling to cope with these emotions, please reach out for help. There are many resources available to help you, such as support groups, therapy, and medication.

Caring for a premature baby can be a challenging experience, but it is also a very rewarding one. By taking care of yourself, you will be better able to care for your baby and help them thrive.

**Some additional tips for self-care:**


*Do something you enjoy*. This could be anything from reading a book to taking a yoga class.

*** Spend time with people who make you feel good**. This could be your partner, family, friends, or support group.

*** Do not be afraid to ask for help**. Your healthcare providers, family, and friends are there to support you.


*Remember, you are not alone. Numerous people are interested in assisting you and care about you.*

# CHAPTER 12

# Resources for parents of premature babies

There are many resources available to parents of premature babies. These resources can provide information, support, and guidance during this challenging time.

Some examples of resources for parents of premature babies include:

1. **Books and websites**: There are many books and websites that provide information about premature birth, NICU care, and parenting a preemie. Some of these resources are written by medical professionals, while others are written by parents who have been through the experience of having a premature baby.

2. **Support groups**: There are many support groups available for parents of premature babies. These groups can provide a safe place

for parents to share their experiences, ask questions, and get support from others who understand what they are going through.

3. **Online forums**: There are also many online forums for parents of premature babies. These forums can be a great way to connect with other parents, ask questions, and get support.

4. **Phone hotlines**:There are also many phone hotlines available for parents of premature babies. These hotlines can provide information, support, and guidance 24 hours a day.

If you are the parent of a premature baby, there are many resources available to help you. Please don't hesitate to reach out for help.

*Here are a few extra assets that you might view as supportive::*

*March of Dimes*: The March of Dimes is a non-profit organization that works to improve the health of babies. They offer a variety of resources for parents of premature babies, including information, support, and advocacy.

*National Center for Children in Poverty*: The National Center for Children in Poverty is a research and policy organization that works to improve the lives of low-income children. They offer a variety of resources for parents of premature babies, including information, support, and financial assistance.

* **Preemie Parents Worldwide**: Preemie Parents Worldwide is a non-profit organization that provides support and resources to parents of premature babies. They offer a variety of resources, including a website, a forum, and a hotline.

## Helping Premature Babies

There are many things that you can do to help premature babies even if you don't have any!

**Support the parents**: Premature birth can be a very stressful experience for parents. You can offer your support by listening to them, providing practical help, and just being there for them.

**Educate yourself**: The more you know about premature birth, the better equipped you will be to help the parents and the baby. There are many resources available to help you learn more about premature birth.

**Donate to organizations that support premature babies**: There are many organizations that provide support and resources to premature babies and their families. You can donate to these organizations to help make a difference in the lives of premature babies.

**Volunteer your time**: There are many ways to volunteer your time to help premature babies. You can volunteer at a hospital, a neonatal intensive care unit (NICU), or a premature birth support group.
By supporting the parents, educating yourself, donating to organizations, and volunteering your time, you can make a difference in the lives of premature babies.

# CONCLUSION

Caring for a premature baby can be a daunting task, but it is also an incredibly rewarding one. With the right information and support, you can provide your little one with the best possible care.

This book has provided you with a comprehensive overview of premature birth and the care of premature babies. You have learned about the different stages of premature development, the challenges that premature babies face, and the ways in which you can help them.

You have also learned about the importance of bonding with your premature baby and the ways in which you can support your baby's development.

The main thing to recall is that you are in good company. There are many resources available to help you care for your premature baby. Your baby's healthcare team is there to support you every step of the way.

With love and support, your premature baby can thrive. They are a tiny miracle, and you are their miracle worker.

Here are some additional tips for caring for your premature baby:

* Get to know your baby's healthcare team. They are there to help you and your baby, so don't be afraid to ask questions.
* Be patient. It may take time for your baby to catch up to their full-term peers.
* Don't compare your baby to other babies. Every baby is different, and your baby is perfect just the way they are.
* Take care of yourself. It's important to take care of your own physical and emotional health so that you can be there for your baby.

Caring for a premature baby can be a challenge, but it is also an incredibly rewarding experience. With love and support, your premature baby can thrive. They are a tiny miracle, and you are their miracle worker.